GW01229682

Pond Fishing with Papa

By

Mike Watts

Copyright © *Mike Watts,* 2024

All Rights Reserved

This book is subject to the condition that no part of this book is to be reproduced, transmitted in any form or means, electronic or mechanical, stored in a retrieval system, photocopied, recorded, scanned, or otherwise. Any of these actions require the proper written permission of the author.

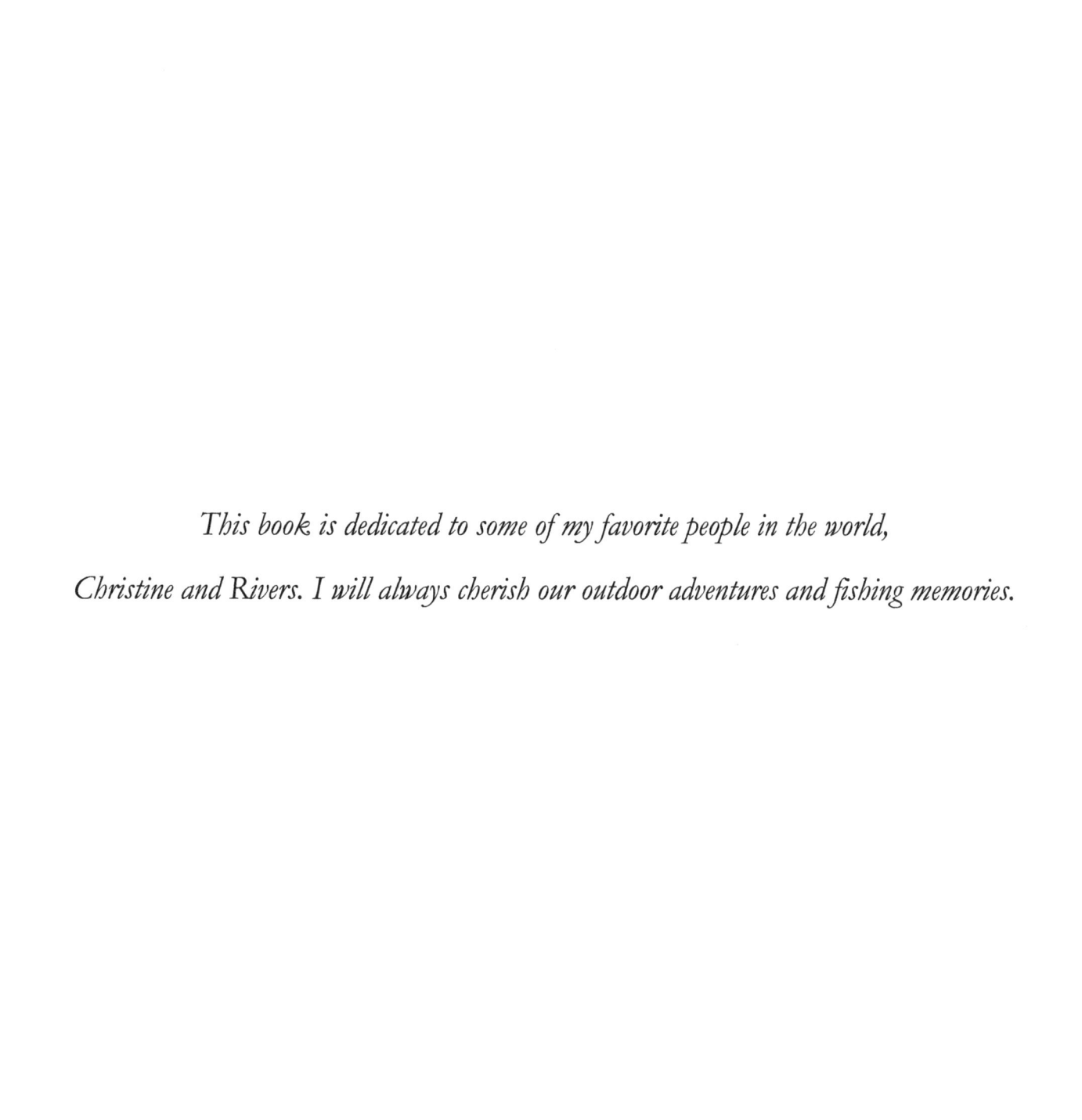

This book is dedicated to some of my favorite people in the world,

Christine and Rivers. I will always cherish our outdoor adventures and fishing memories.

Introduction

"The name Papa, sometimes called Grandpa or Grandad, comes with a rather large obligation. This responsibility includes spoiling the child, sharing great stories of which only tiny parts of it may be true, being able to communicate family history, and explaining the way life used to be when you were a boy. At the same time, this obligation allows Papa the opportunity to look at nature and its intrinsic gifts once again through the eyes of a child."

"I embraced this job description and began fulfilling it several years ago. I started by taking my grandson, Rivers, fishing, always making it less about the fish and more about our time together. And while I am never too old to drown worms with my grandson in a farm pond, I always have a fly rod within arm's reach."[1]

This book was originally the idea of my daughter, Christine, a mom herself, who encouraged me to share my passion for fishing through the writing of children's books. She collaborated her thoughts and ideas with mine, and the stories developed. The stories reflect many first-hand experiences, such as taking my daughter and grandson fishing as children. Each of the stories has been field-tested and approved by a six-year-old.

We aim to create a series of "Fishing with Papa" books covering different species and techniques and introducing children to the outdoors and various types of fishing.

---

[1] "Rivers and the Great Trout" by Mike Watts   published in South Carolina Wildlife magazine September-October issue 2023

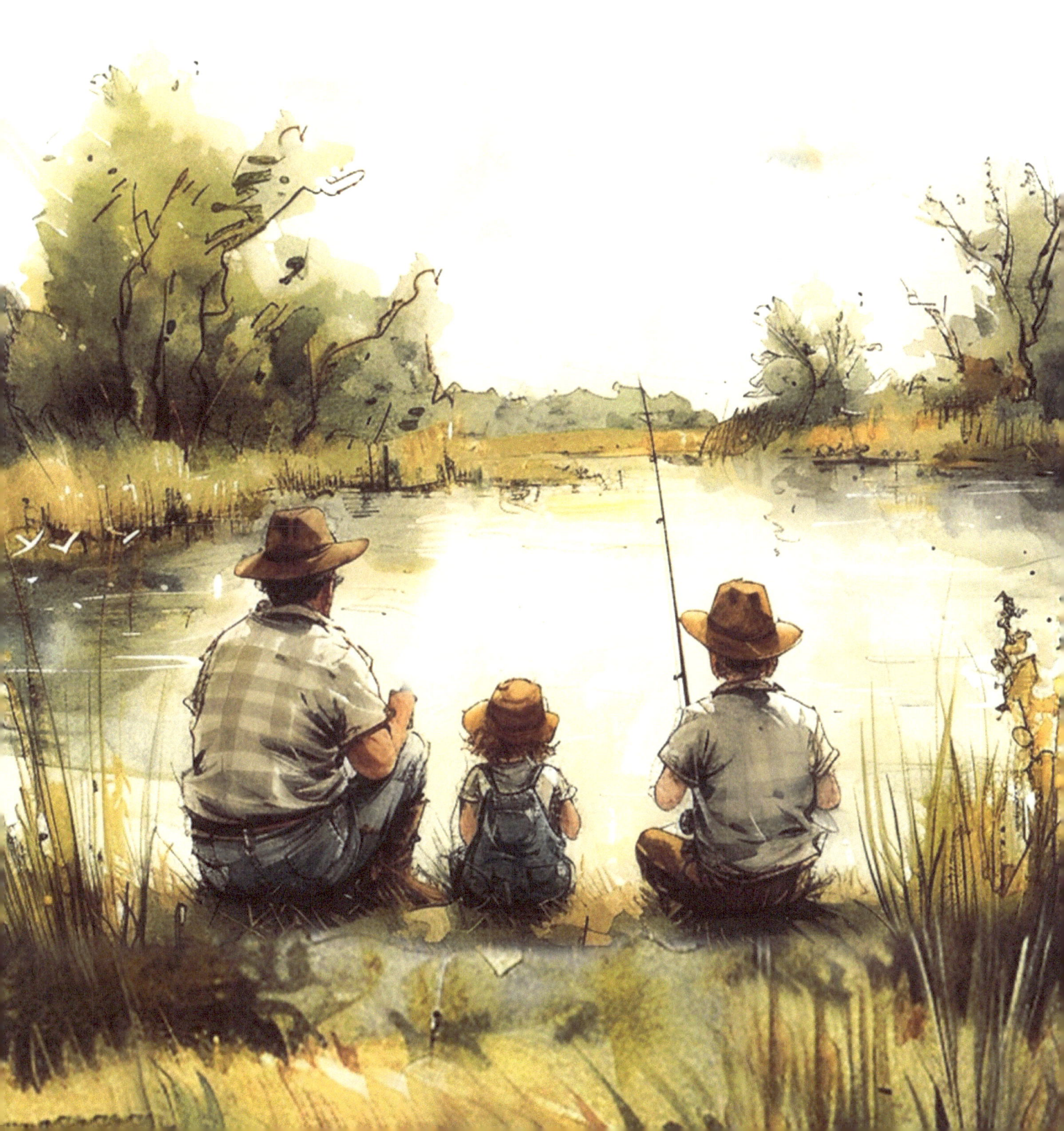

My little brother Andy and I always loved visiting our grandparents' farm in the mountains of north Georgia. They made every visit special for us. Papa could always be counted on to make us laugh and giggle with his fishing stories.

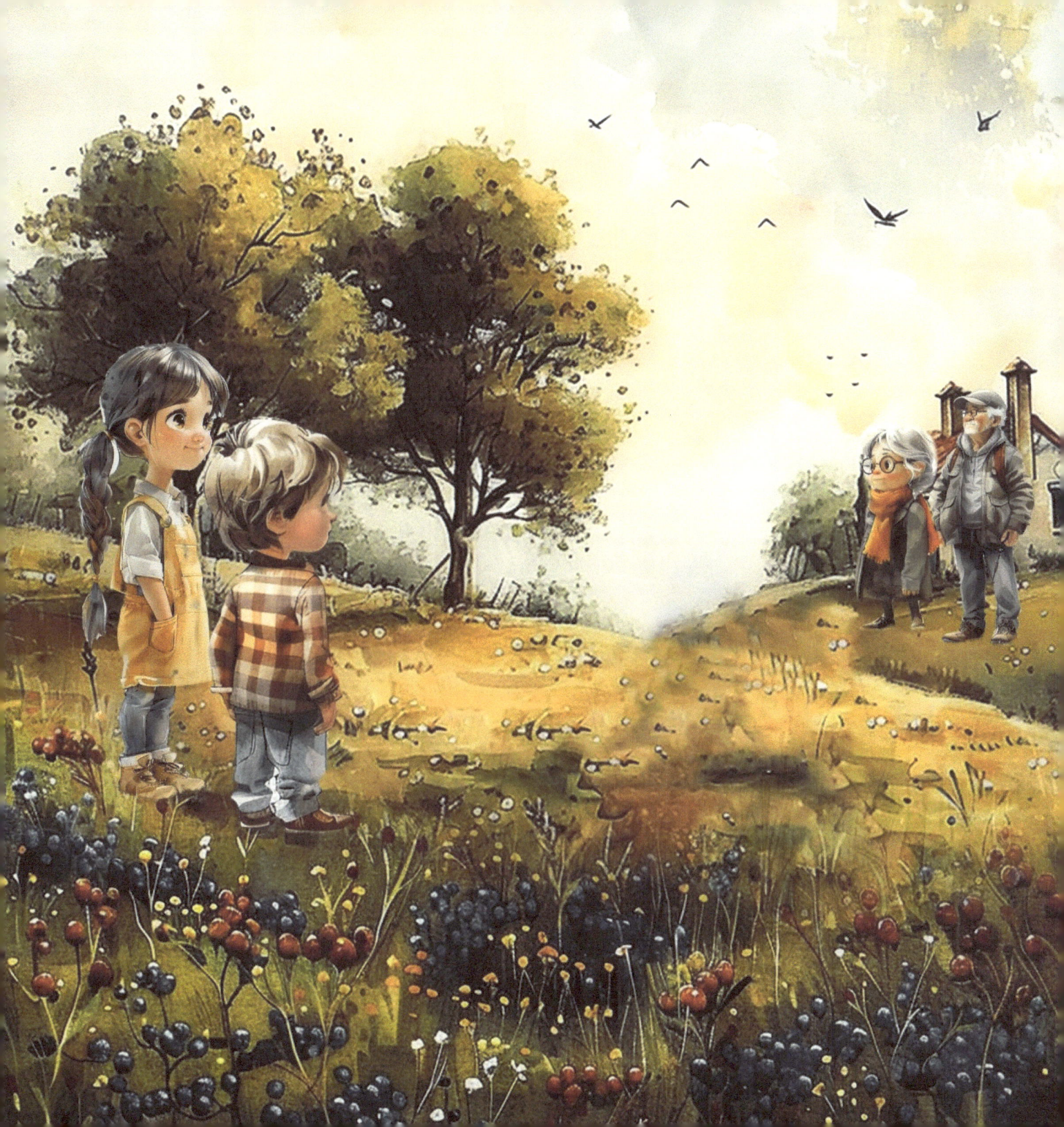

At dinner on the first night, Papa said, "Sally, I'll wake you and Andy before daylight to go fishing. Today, I met a great blue heron tiptoeing around the pond's edge, and the heron told me the fish were biting at daylight."

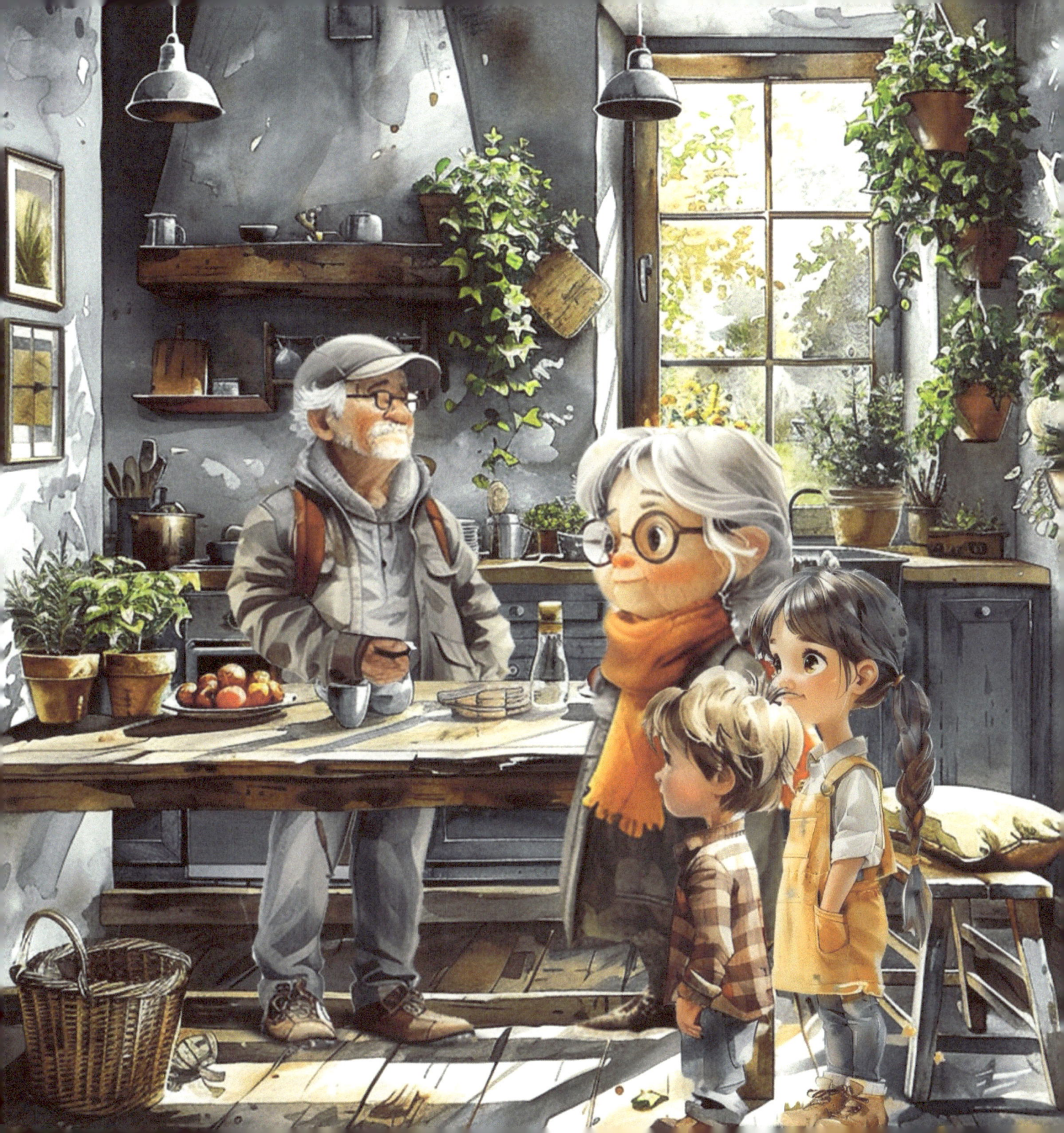

Of course, we didn't believe him. I told Papa that birds couldn't talk, and Andy agreed. Then we laughed as Papa stood up and began tiptoeing around the dining room like a heron. He lifted each leg slowly forward and silently placed it back toe first, careful not to splash water or spook any fish. Papa told us always to pay attention to nature and that we could learn new things just by watching the wildlife.

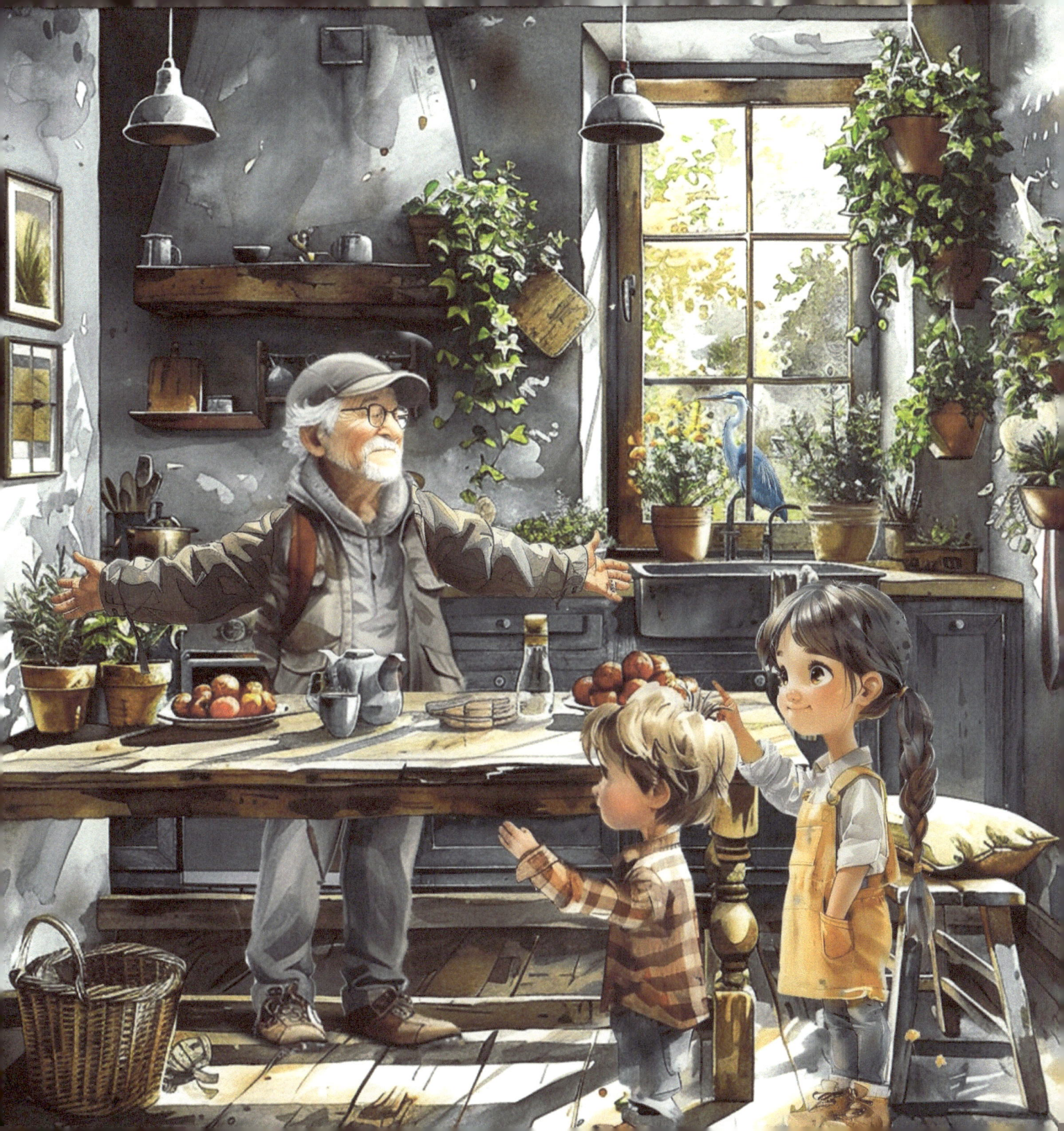

The next morning came quickly. We woke up to the smell of bacon frying and could hear Mimi cracking eggs on the countertop. It was still dark when Papa met us at the back door, ready to leave.

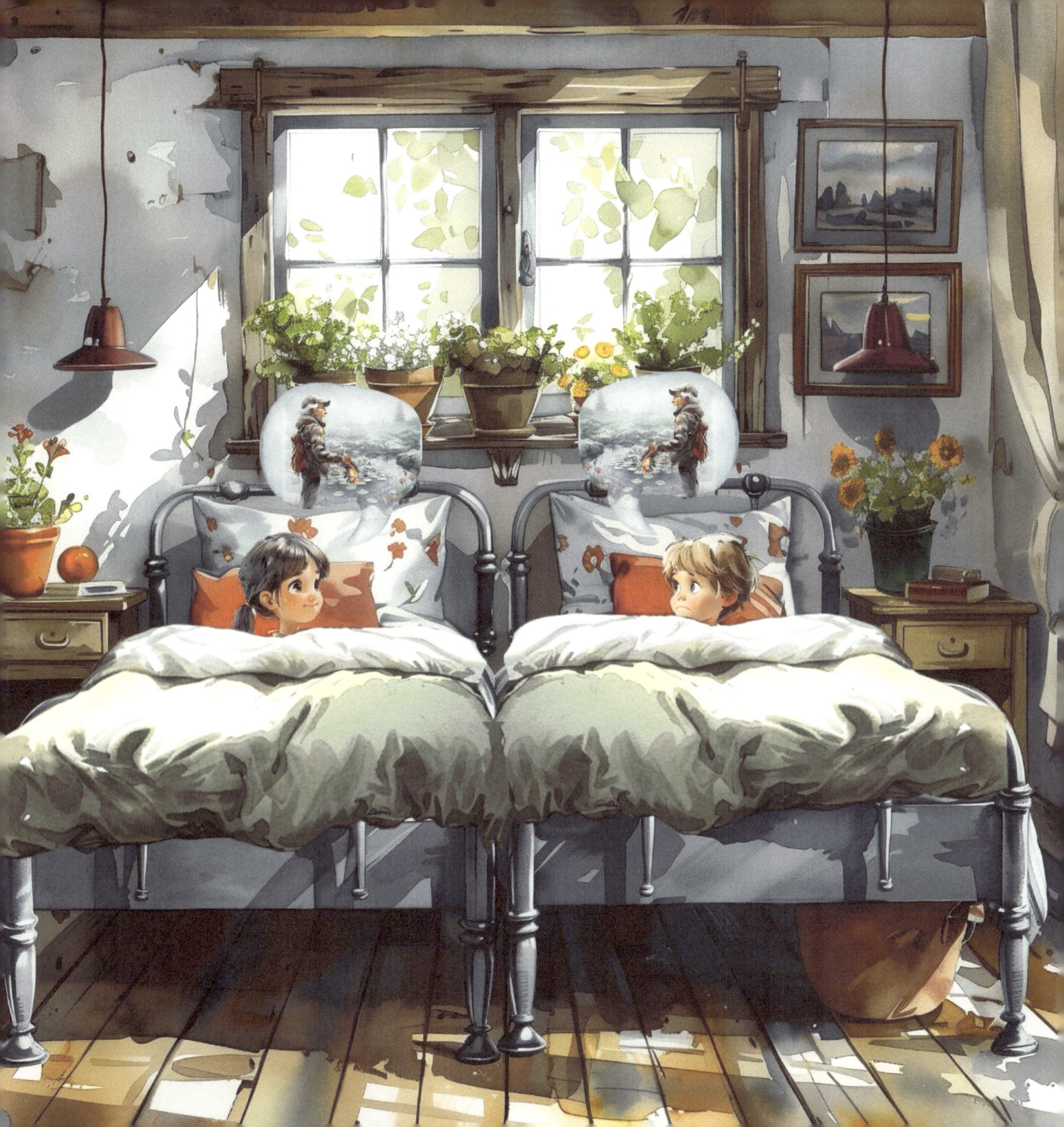

He handed us each a fishing rod to carry. He thought I was responsible enough to carry his rusty tackle box, which he called the "magic fishing box." Papa said he could always find exactly what he was looking for when he opened it. Every time I shook the box, it sounded like loose nuts and bolts inside a plastic cup. Papa heard me, smiled, bent down, and told me, "What you hear may not always be what it sounds like!"

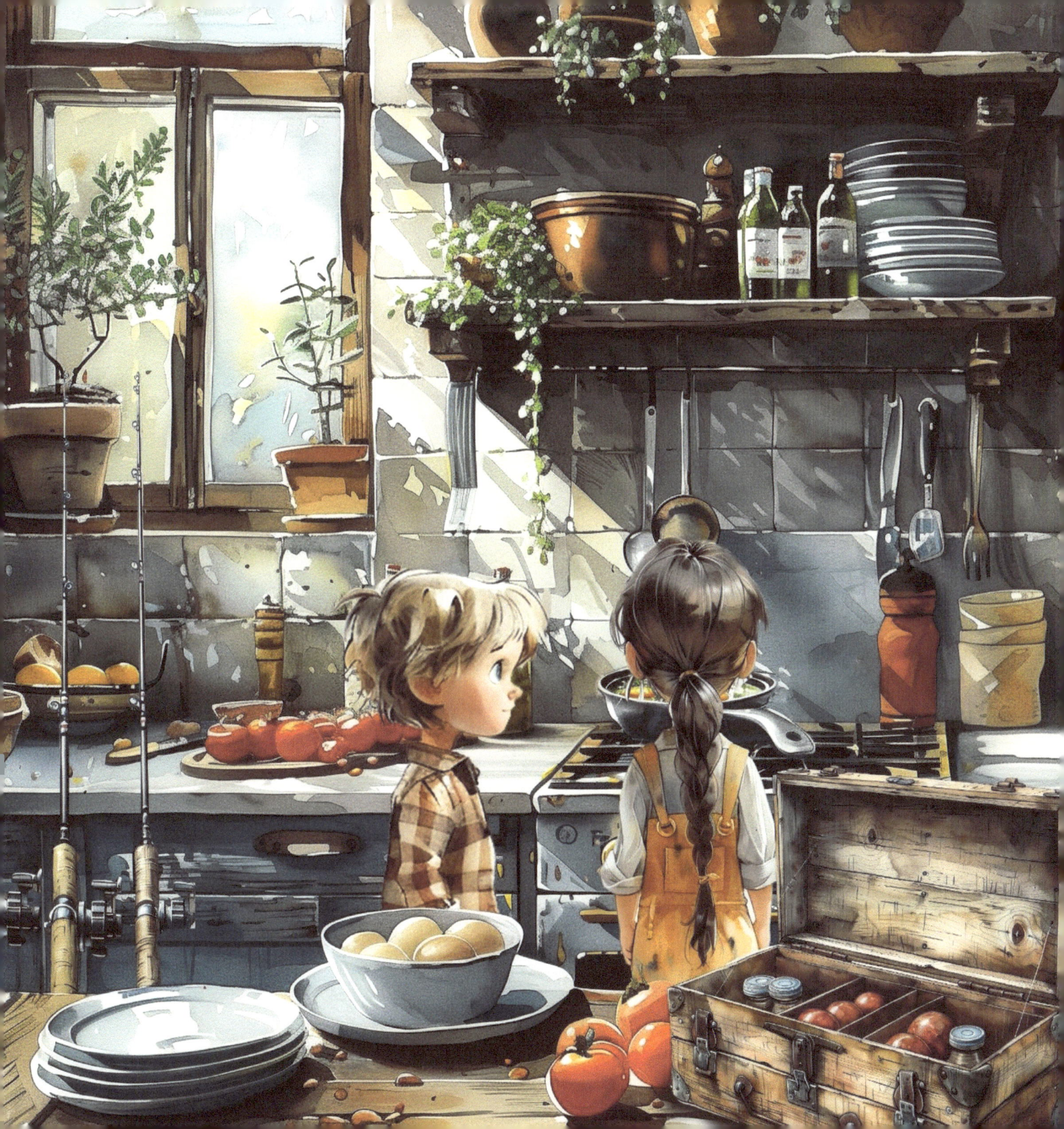

As we walked briskly down the path to the pond, he told us to hurry. He said, "Sunrise only happens once daily, and we didn't want to miss it." The sun started peeping over the mountain as we approached the little dock where Papa tied his boat.

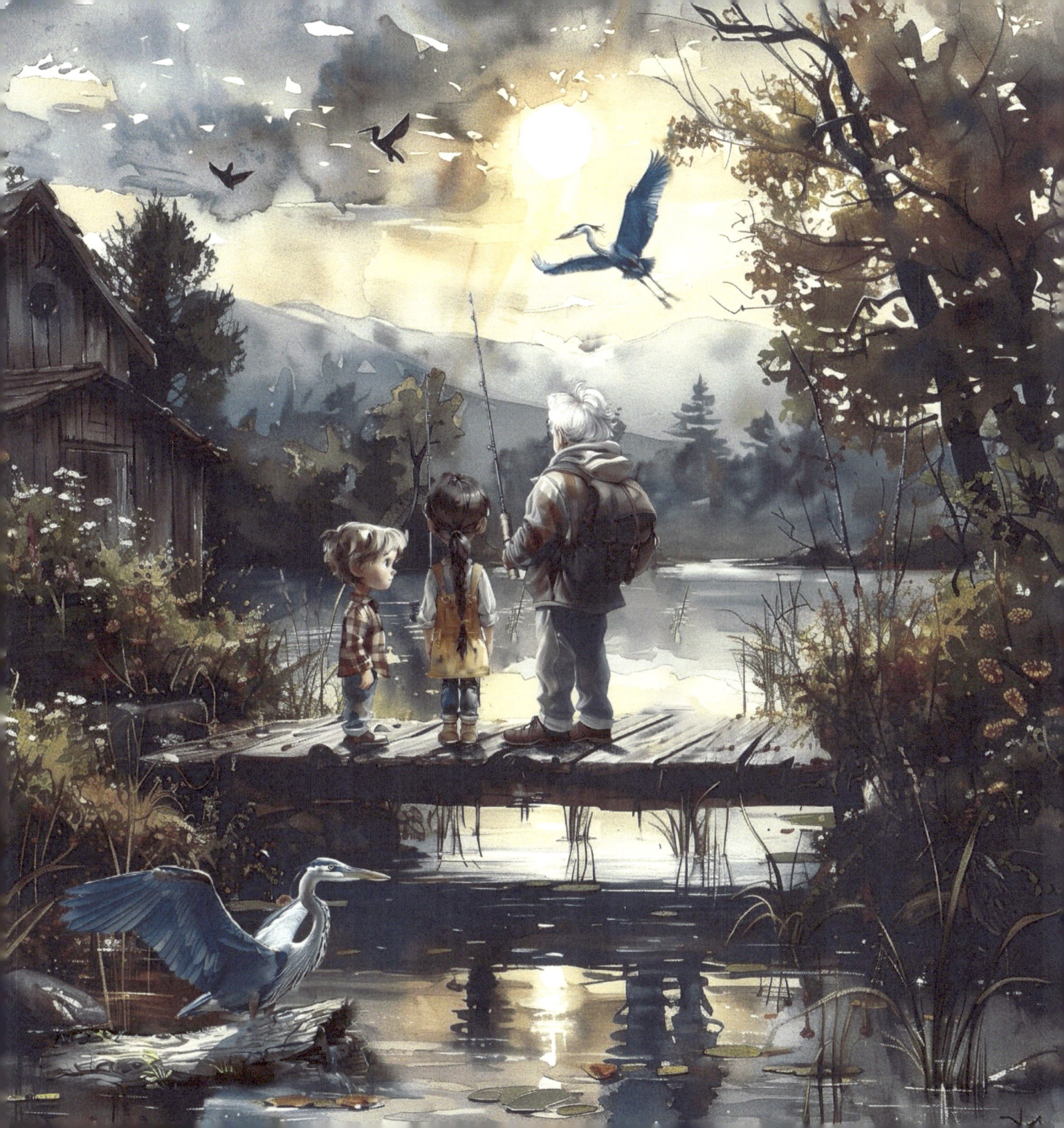

Before we stepped into the boat, he told us to listen quietly. He could hear fish calling our names, but we needed to be quiet to hear them. We didn't hear any fish talking but heard several bullfrogs belching from the high grass along the shoreline and saw songbirds waking up and flitting around the bushes. Suddenly, a heron flew into the pond, squawking loudly as it landed on a log nearby.

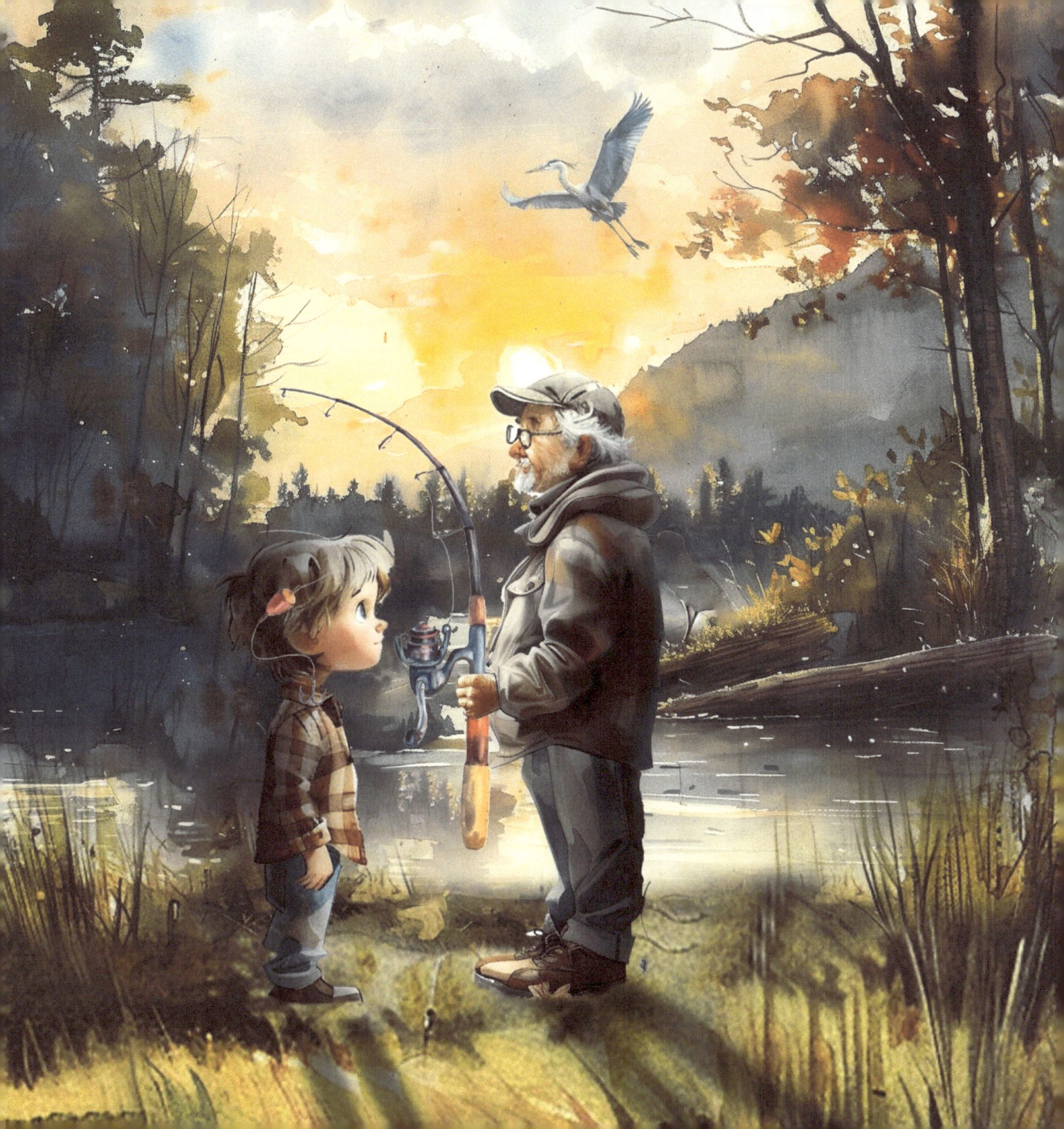

"It's time to go fishing," he said. The water was so peaceful and still, except for the ripples made by Papa quietly paddling the boat. I could see the reflection of all the trees and mountaintops in the water. We watched the heron move around the shoreline, searching for a meal, and we giggled about how clumsy Papa looked while mimicking it.

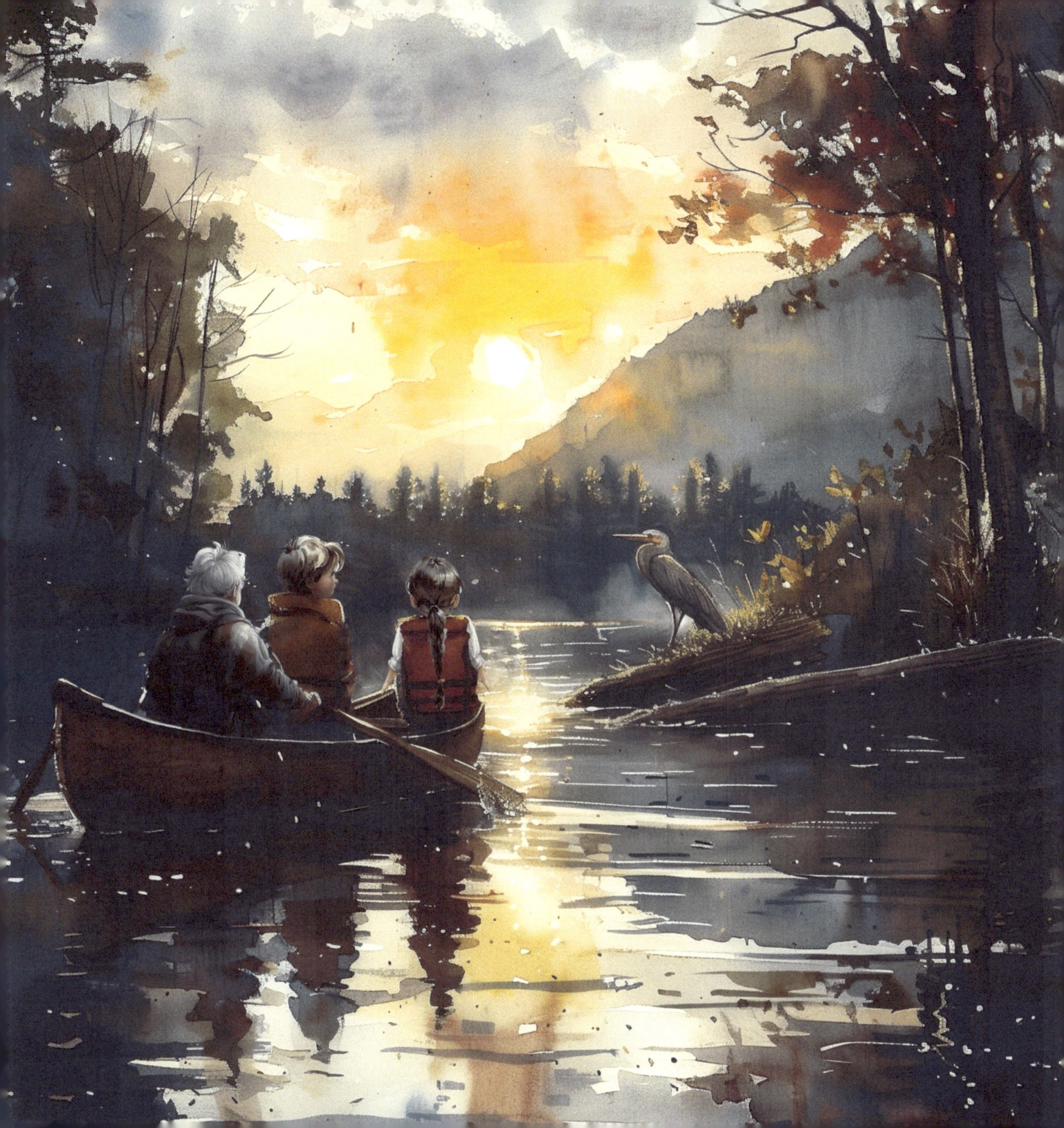

He told Andy he would use "jumping" crickets to catch bream, sometimes called "sunfish." He tried to fool us into thinking he ate a cricket before baiting Andy's hook. But we knew better.

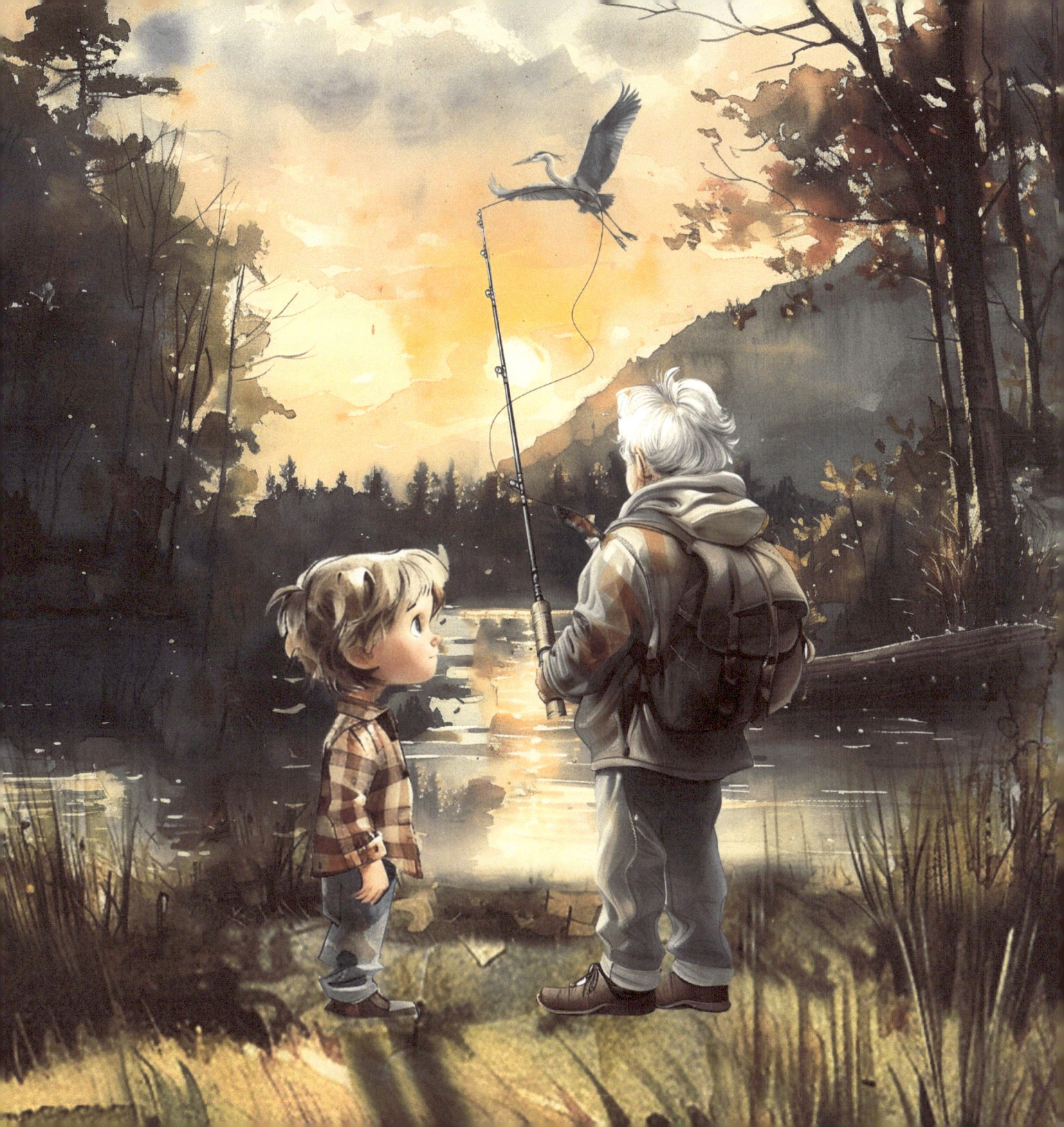

The spinning rods were rigged with a red and white bobber and a small hook to hold the bait. He threw Andy's line out just a few feet from the boat's right edge and told him to lift the rod and pull back if the cork went underwater.

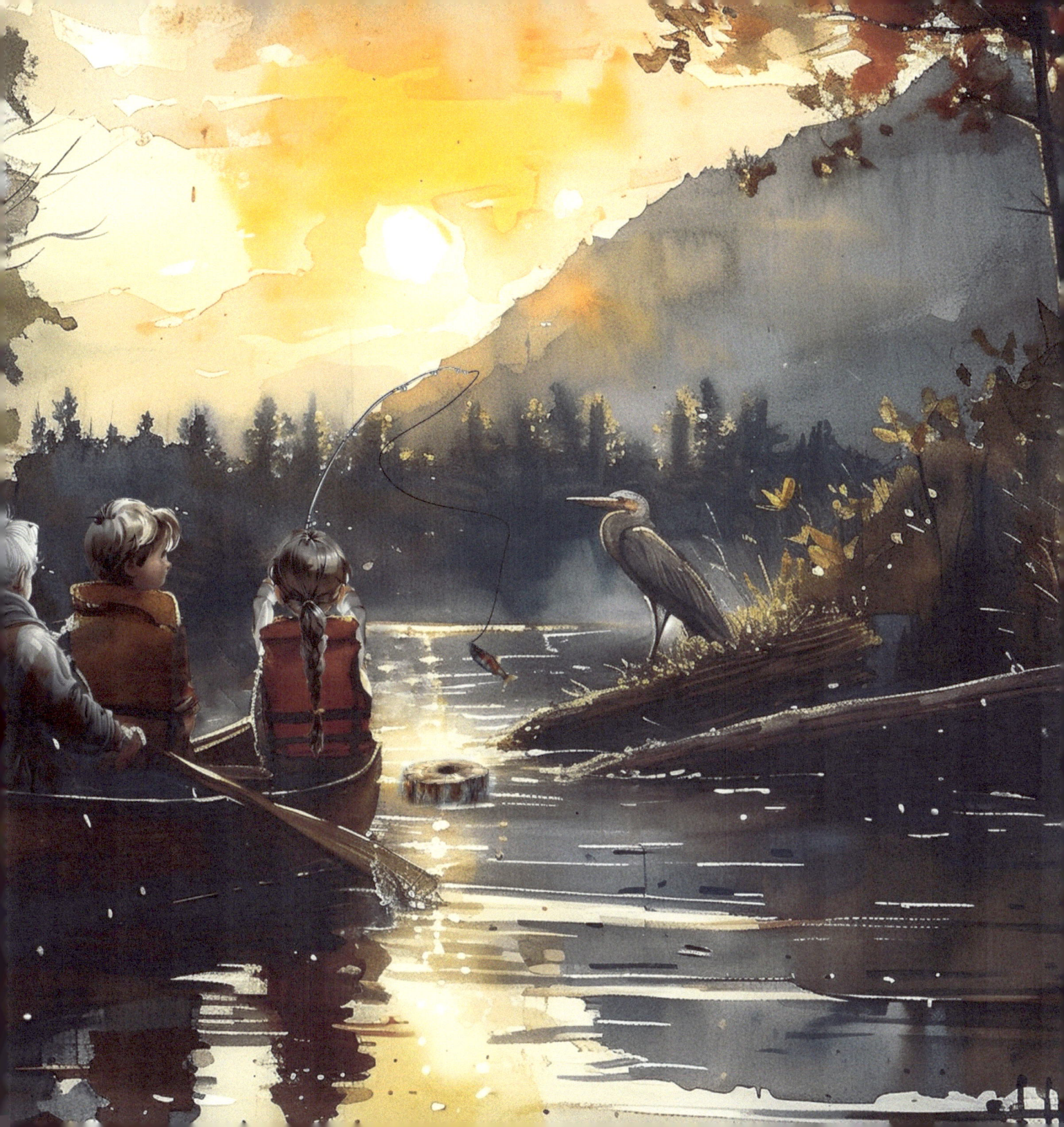

Meanwhile, he grabbed another spinning rod, pulled out a minnow bucket full of "special minnows," and told me to stick my hand in there and spread my fingers apart. The minnows tickled as they swam through my fingers. When I pulled my hands from the water, I noticed tiny, sparkling fish scales stuck between my fingers. Papa called it minnow dust and told me it was more powerful than fairy dust, and if I made a wish about catching a big fish, it would probably come true.

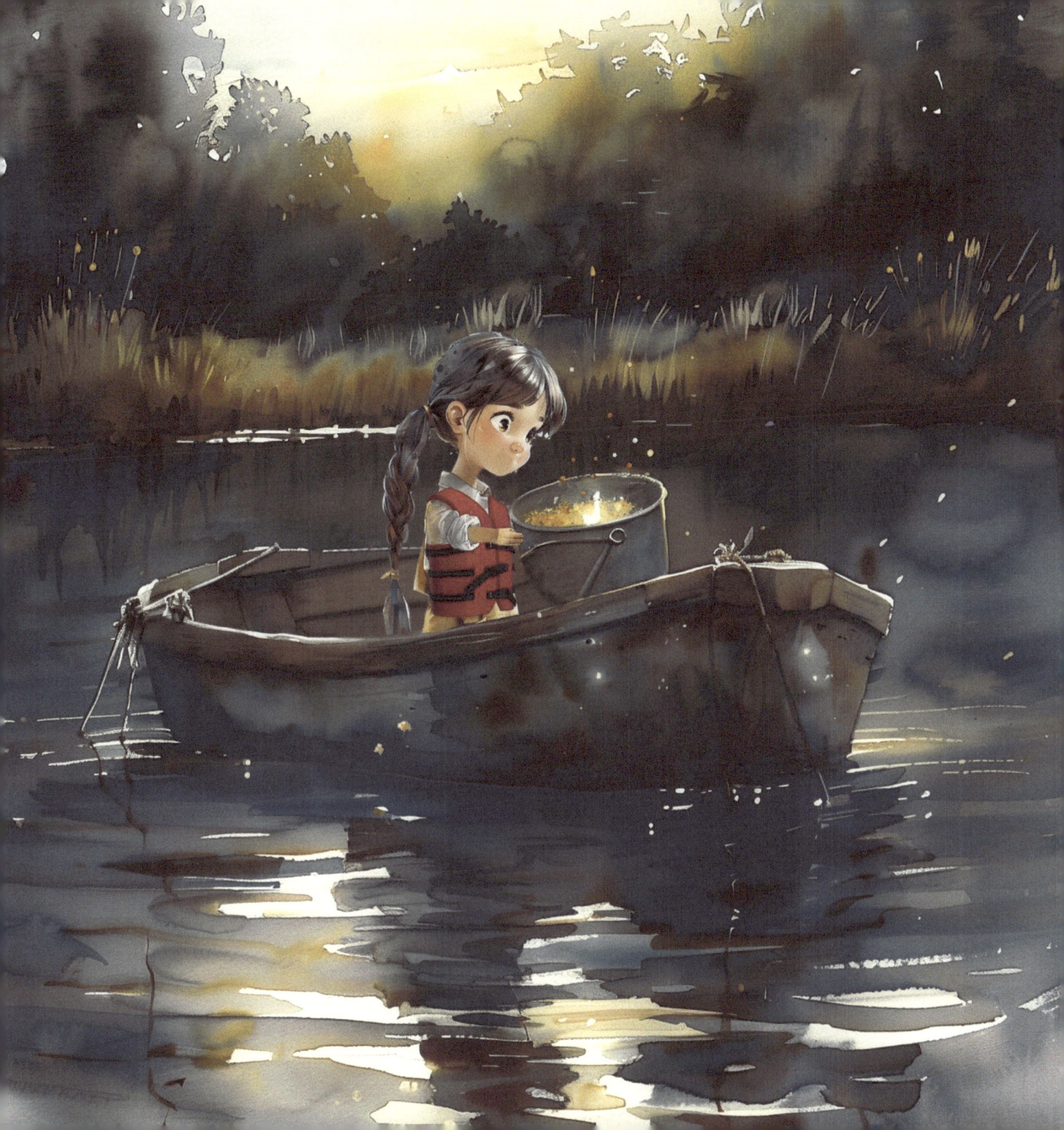

He baited my hook and cast the rod to the other side of the boat, landing it next to a brush pile sticking up from the water's surface. I imagined this brush pile as a tiny jungle island full of tree limbs, sticks, and hidden creatures. I hoped below the water's surface was a cave holding a big, hungry fish that would eat my minnow for breakfast.

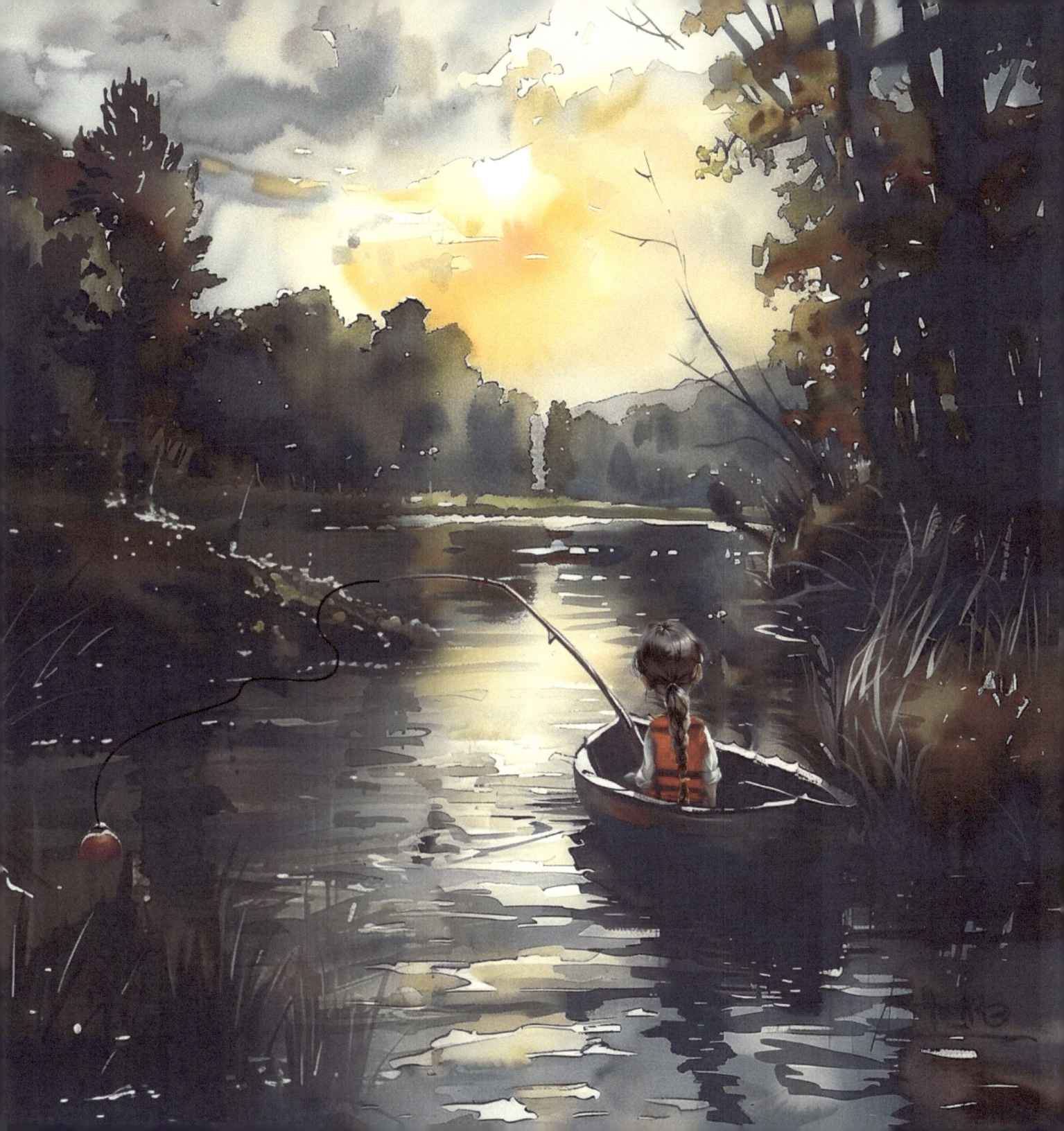

It wasn't long before Andy's bobber disappeared below the water's surface. Andy quickly grabbed the rod, and Papa told him to lift the rod tip. Papa instructed him not to turn the reel handle when the fish pulled hard and swam away. Even with Andy's excitement, he listened to Papa.

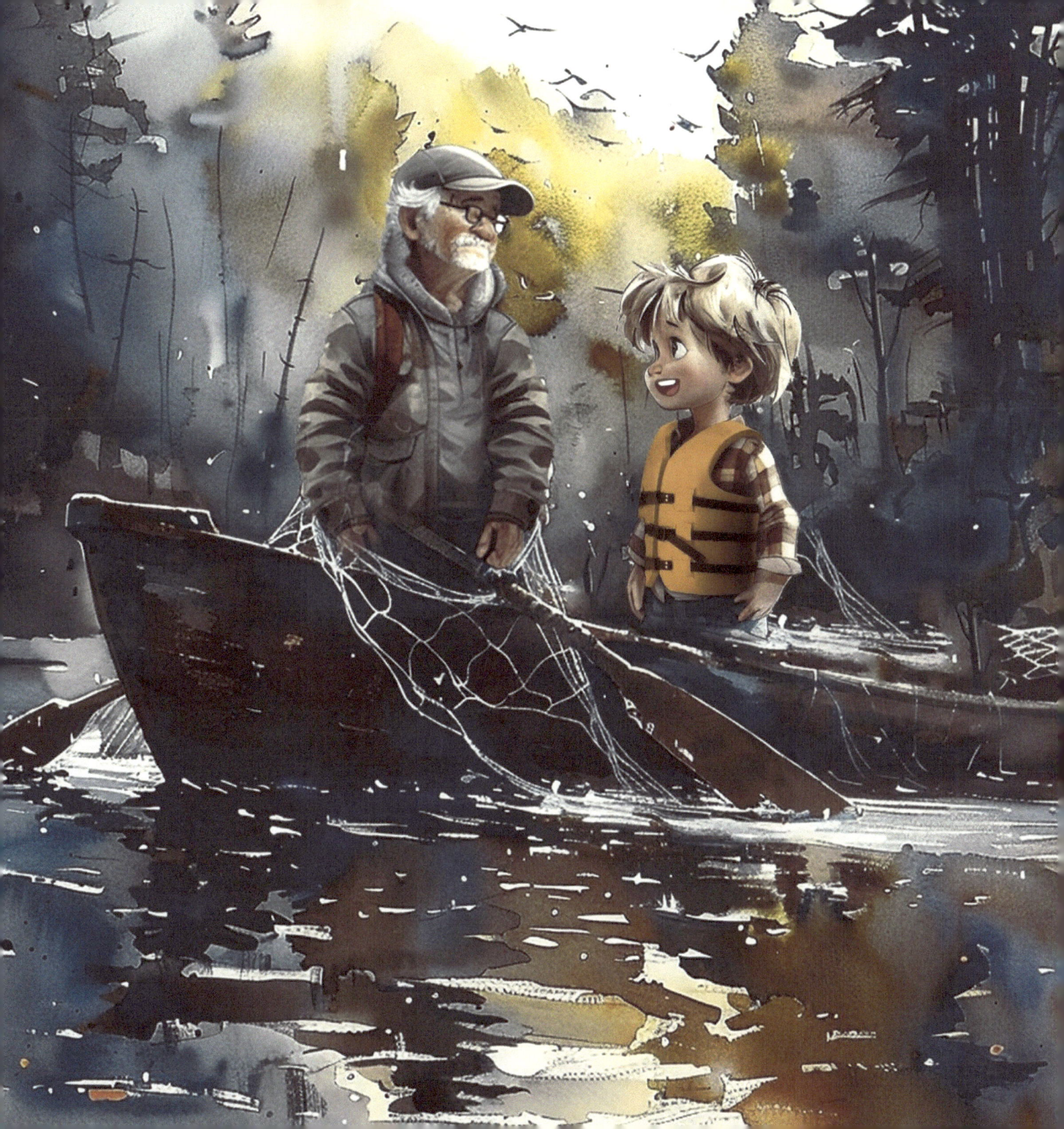

Andy fought the fish as it tried to pull the rod tip underwater, darting back and forth, causing the bobber to sink and pop up. Andy was focused as the fish swam from one end of the boat to the other. I saw him gritting his teeth when he turned the reel handle and grinning as the fish continued to get closer. Finally, the fish was netted and brought into the boat for us all to see.

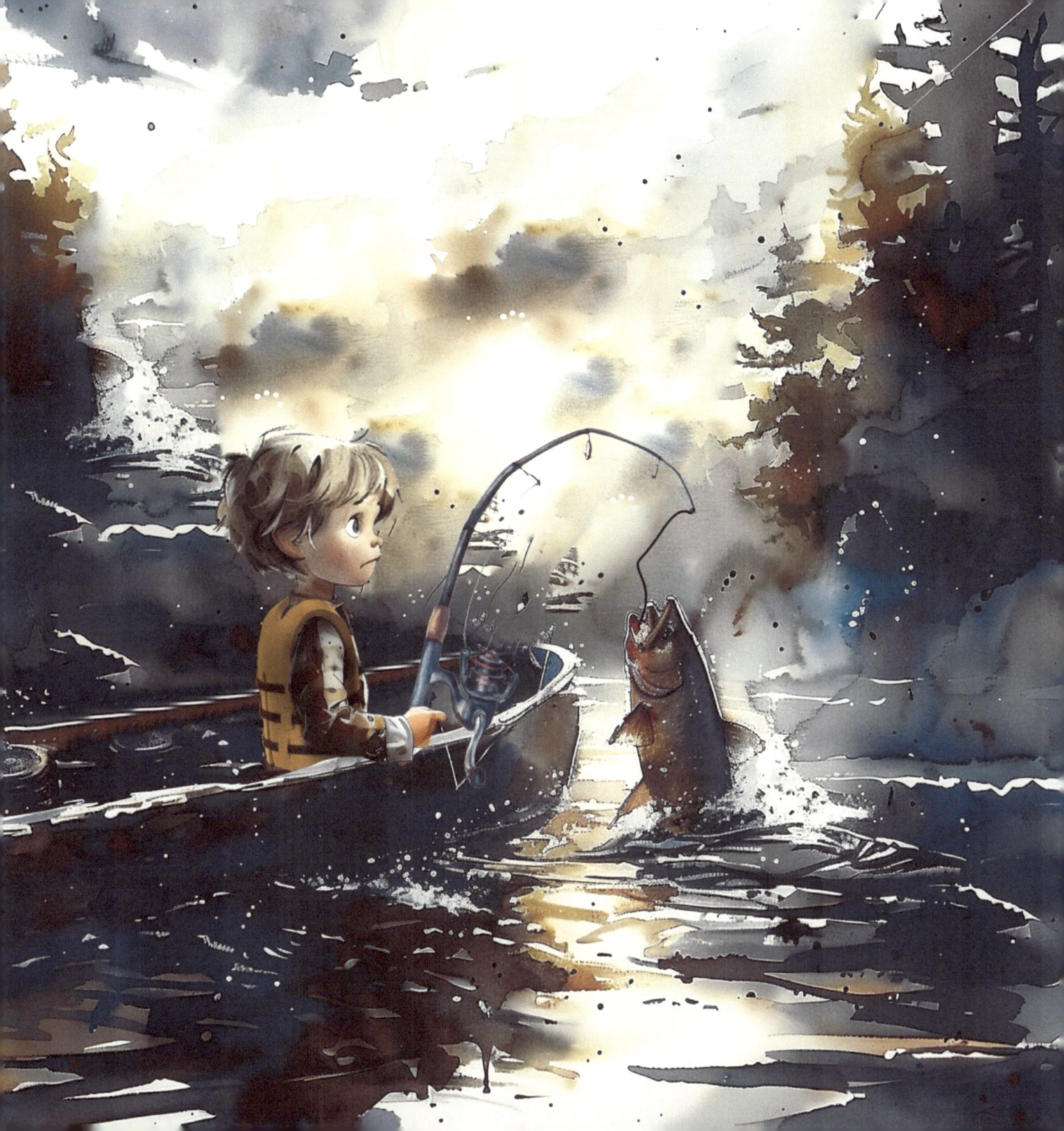

Andy was so proud of his bream. It was bigger than Papa's hands. Papa took it off the hook and gently handed the prized fish back to Andy when it flopped and landed back into the water. We all laughed loudly and teased each other about the fish. Andy insisted Papa rebait his hook with another feisty cricket.

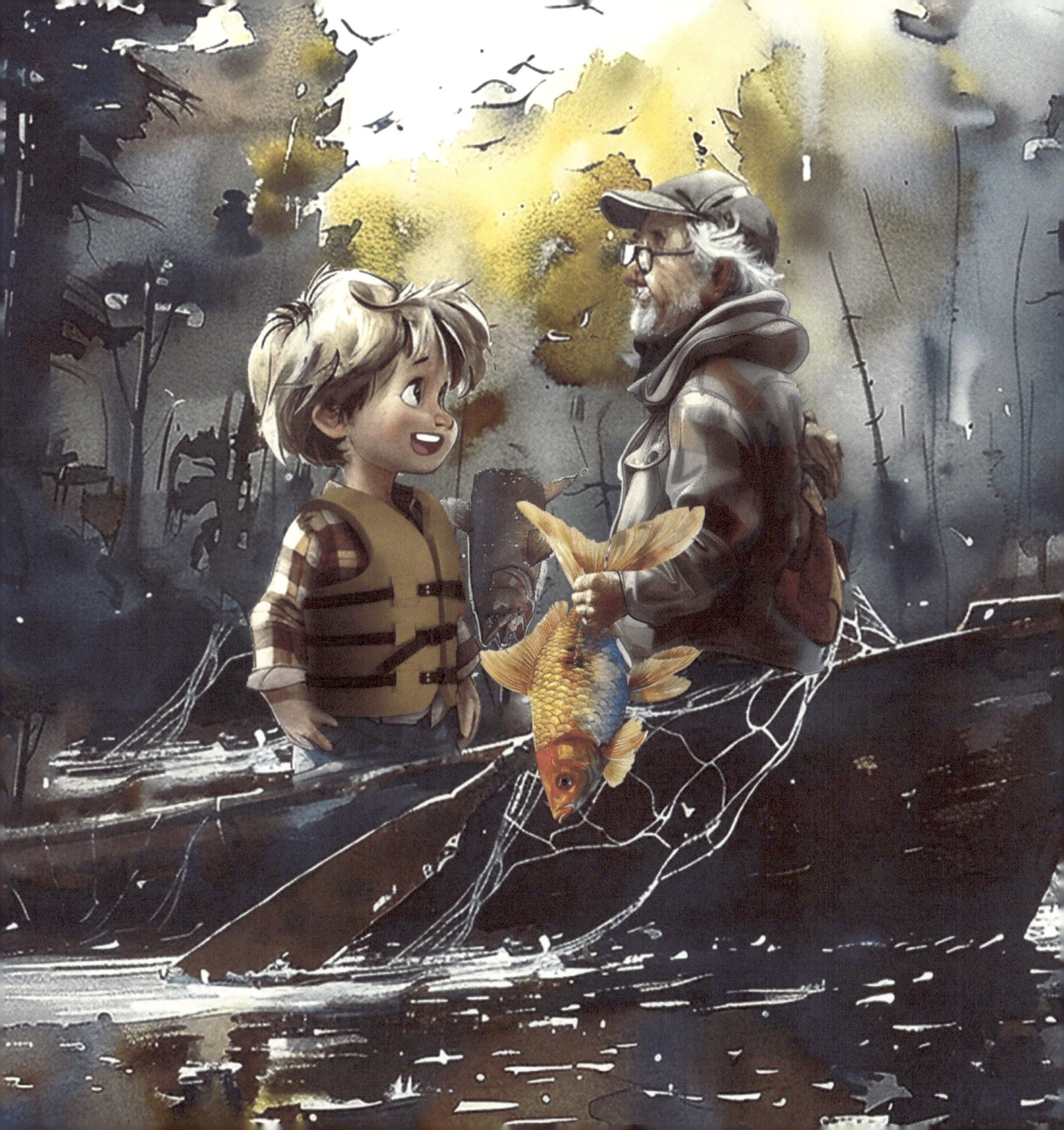

Meanwhile, I had forgotten about my "special" minnow swimming behind me. I glanced over and noticed the bobber slowly moving away from the brush pile. Papa saw it, too. He told me to gently pick up the rod and point the tip towards the bobber. I started to get nervous and tense. I didn't know what to do except to listen to Papa. My hands were shaking with excitement.

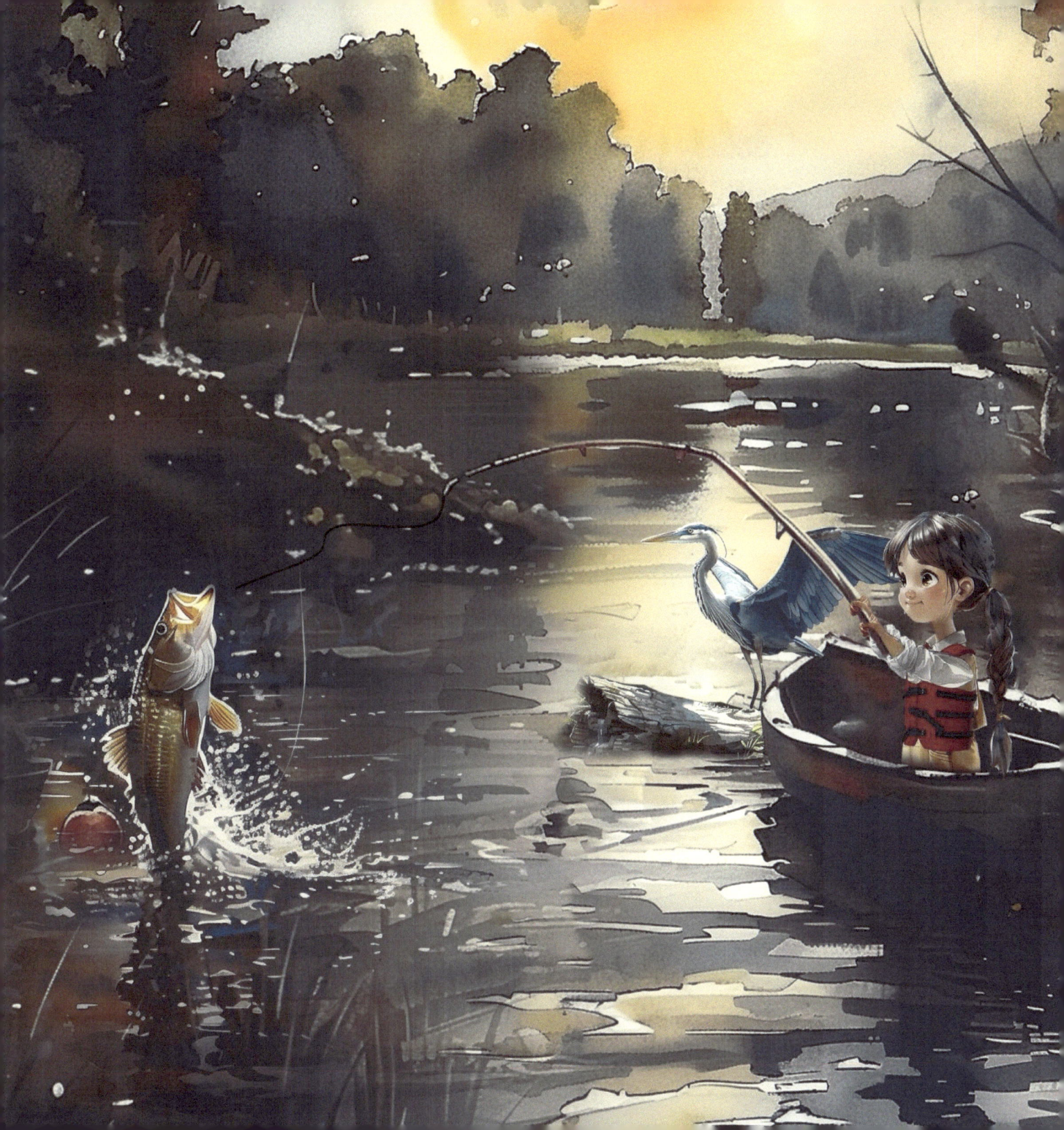

He told me to pull the rod tip up hard as the cork disappeared and hang on. When I did, the fish exploded to the surface and splashed, almost scaring me. I had never seen a fish jump, and I screamed. Andy was laughing at me, but I didn't care. Papa exclaimed, "What a big bass you have hooked there!"

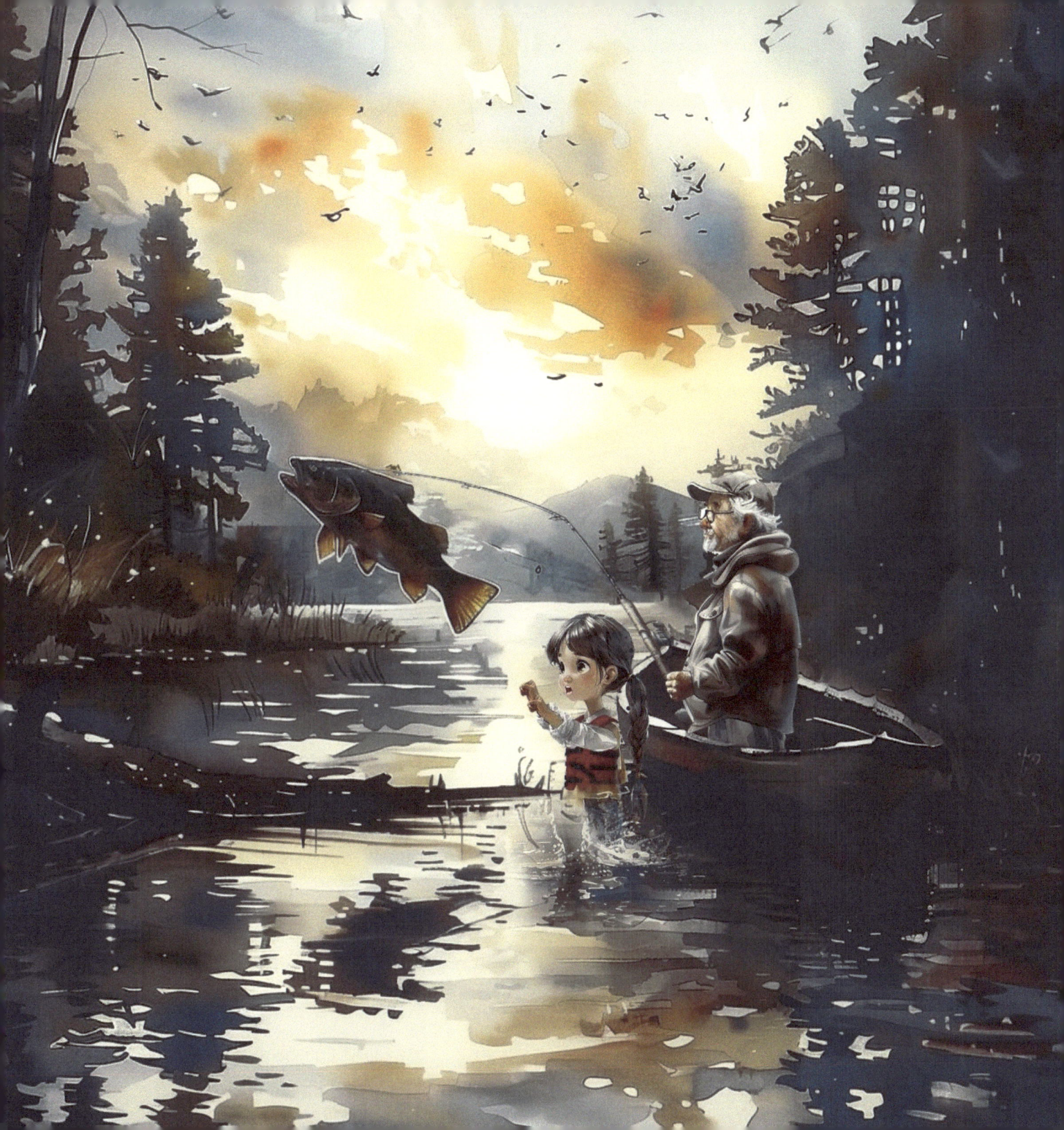

When the bass swam away towards the middle of the pond, Papa reminded me not to turn the reel handle except when the fish was swimming towards me. My arm muscles tightened as I readied myself for battle. This was so much fun. I couldn't control the fish. It tried all kinds of tricks to get away. The fighting fish jerked the rod tip to the left and right, tried pulling it straight out of my hands, and then jumped again.

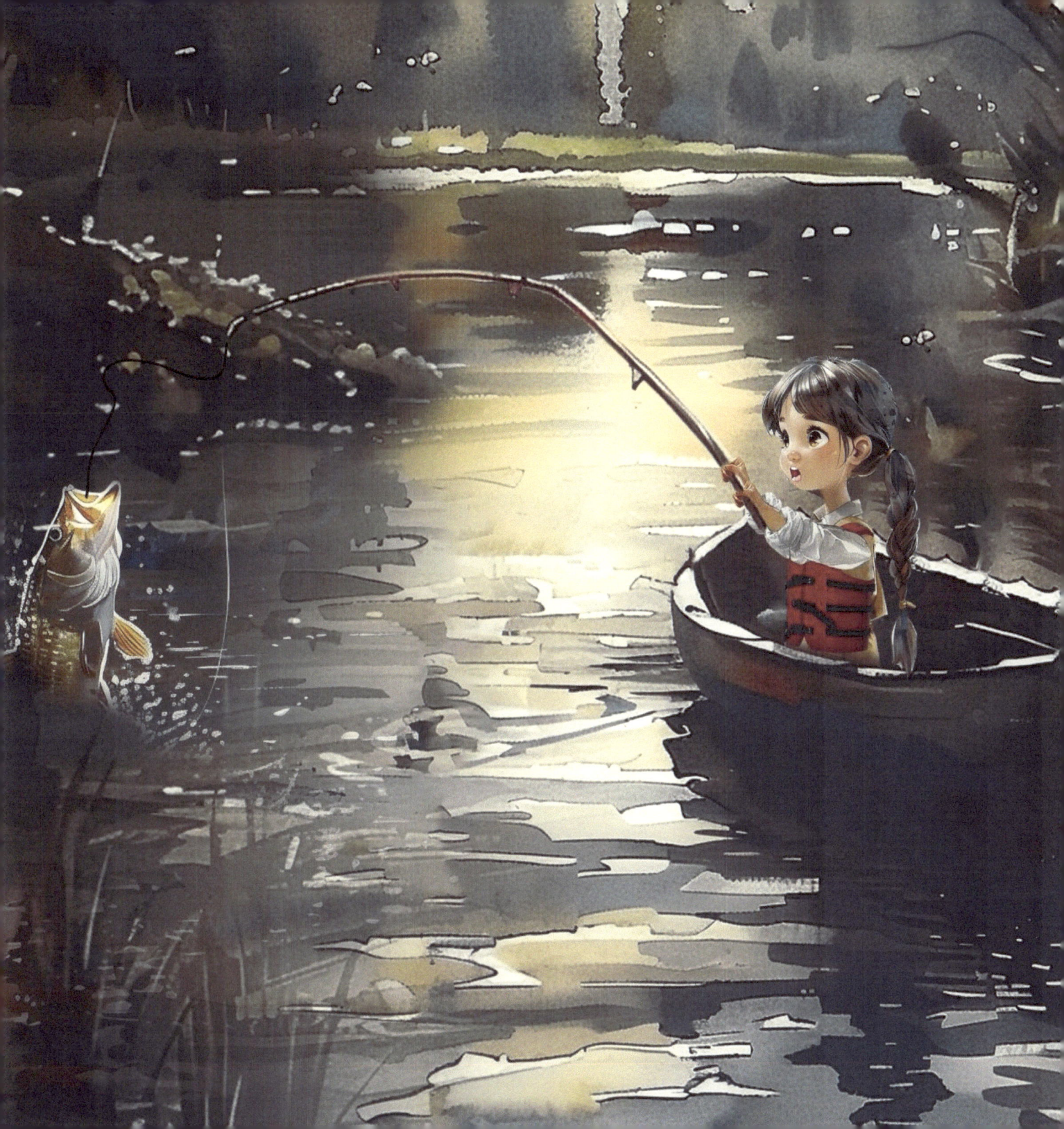

I couldn't believe how hard the fish pulled and how the rod could bend and not break. Finally, as my arms were getting tired, so was the fish. With a little extra rod pressure now, the bass started swimming to the boat, and I reeled it to me. Papa reached down and netted my prize fish.

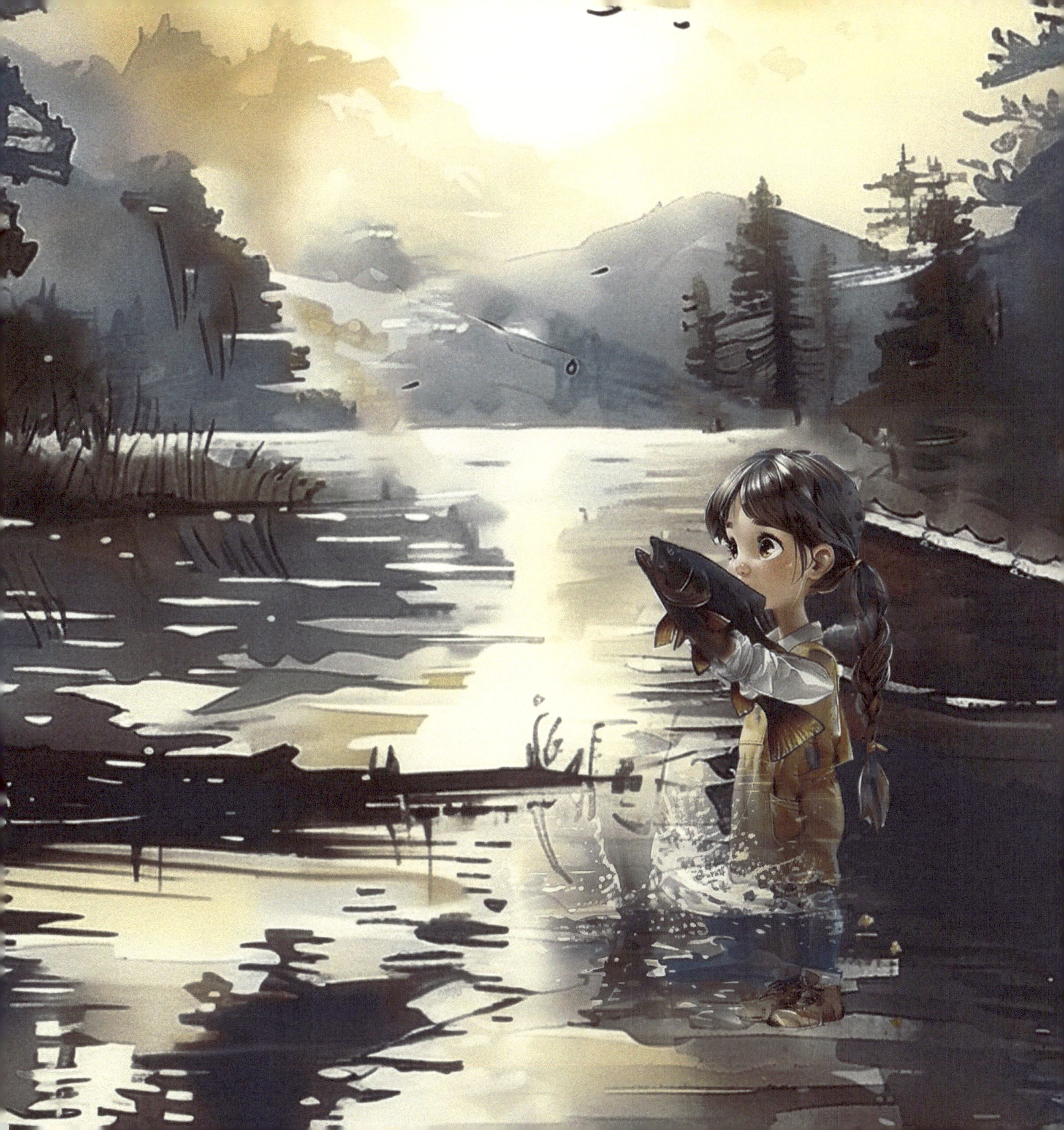

Papa unhooked the bass and had me hold it up. It was so heavy, long, and beautifully green in color along its back. Then he helped me lean over and hold the bass in the water for a minute, and we watched it swim away, ready to be caught again on another visit! I will always remember my goosebumps while fighting my first largemouth bass.

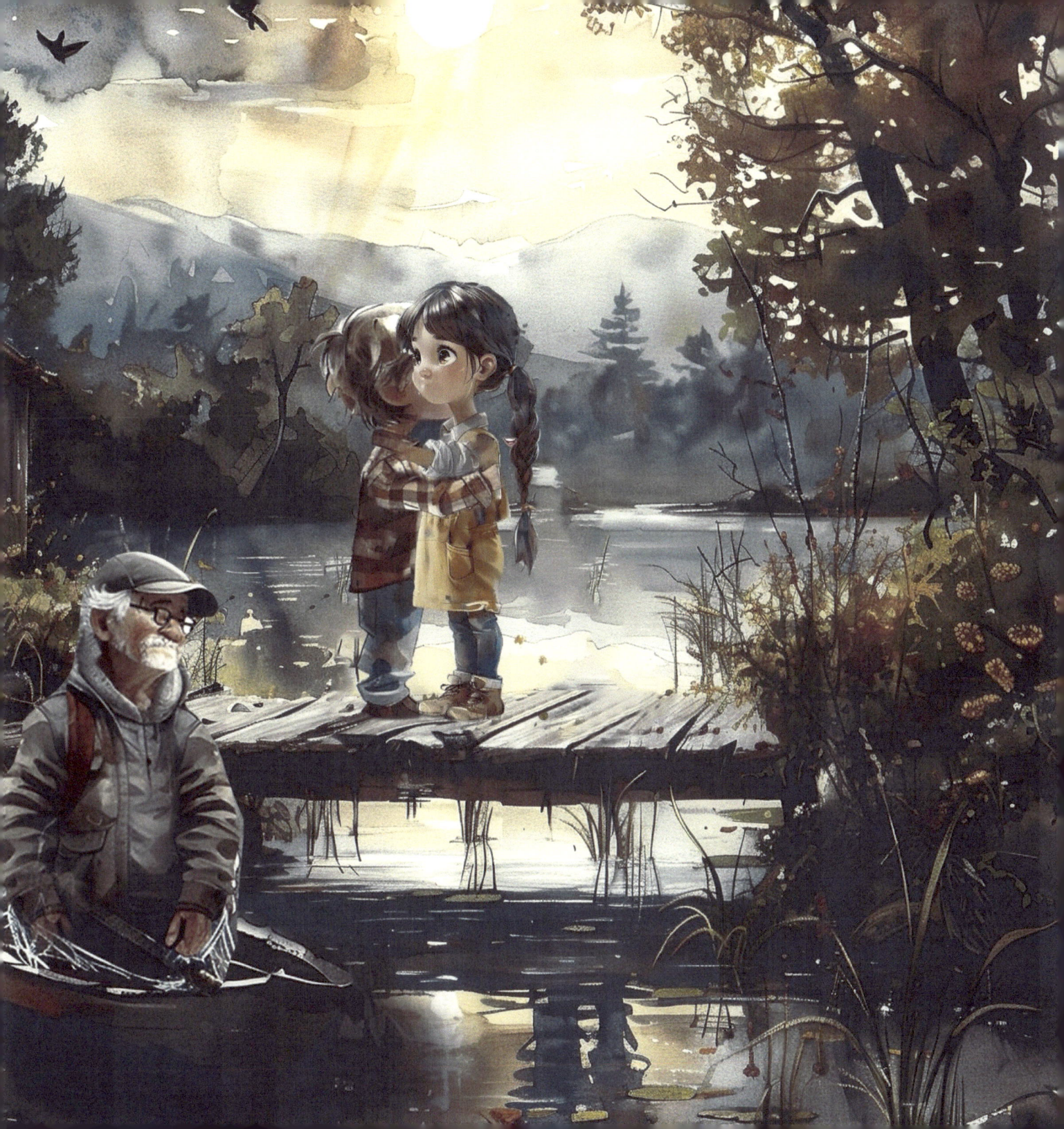

A big fish was living in the brush-piled island after all! Papa was right; fish were calling our name.

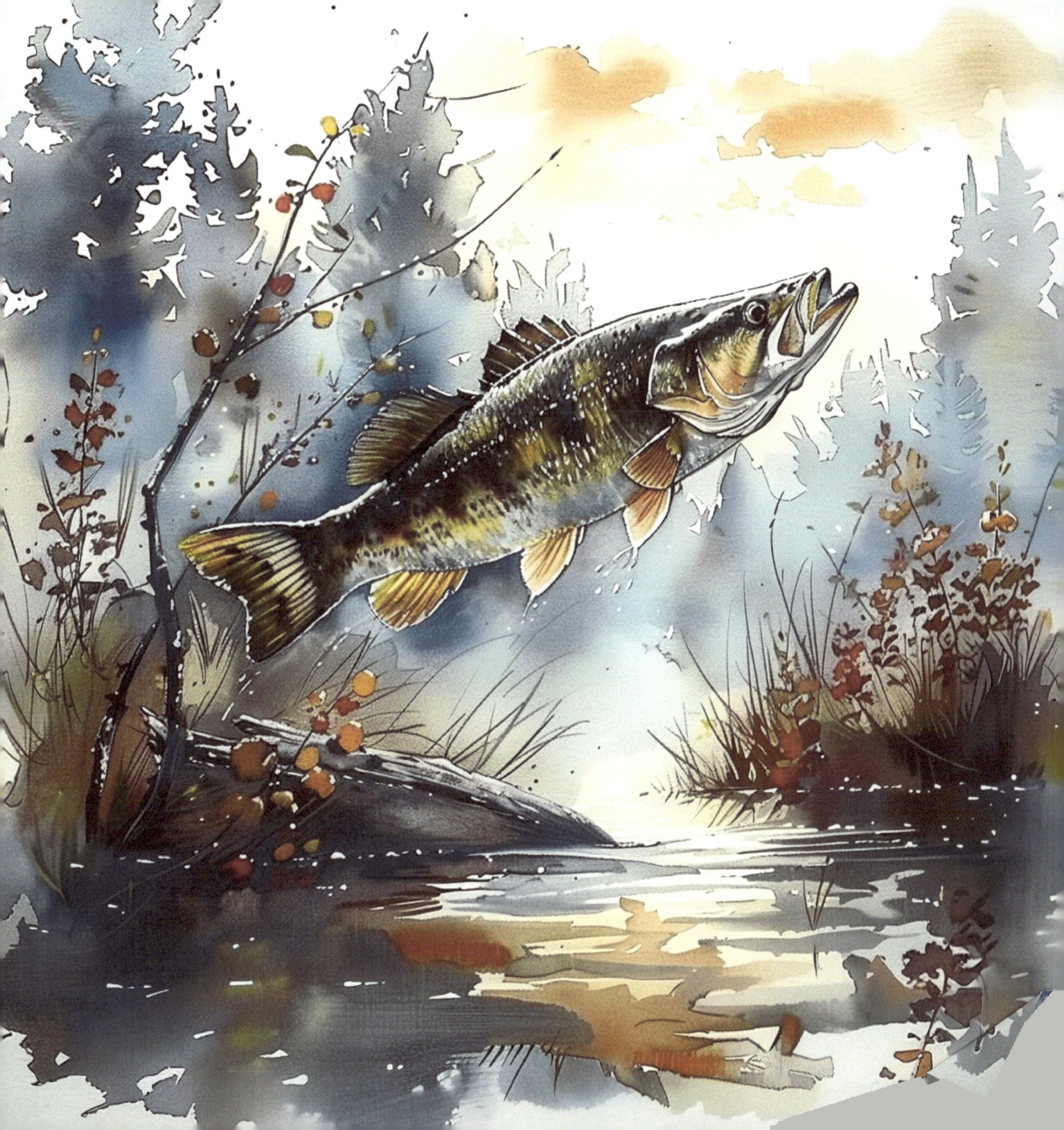

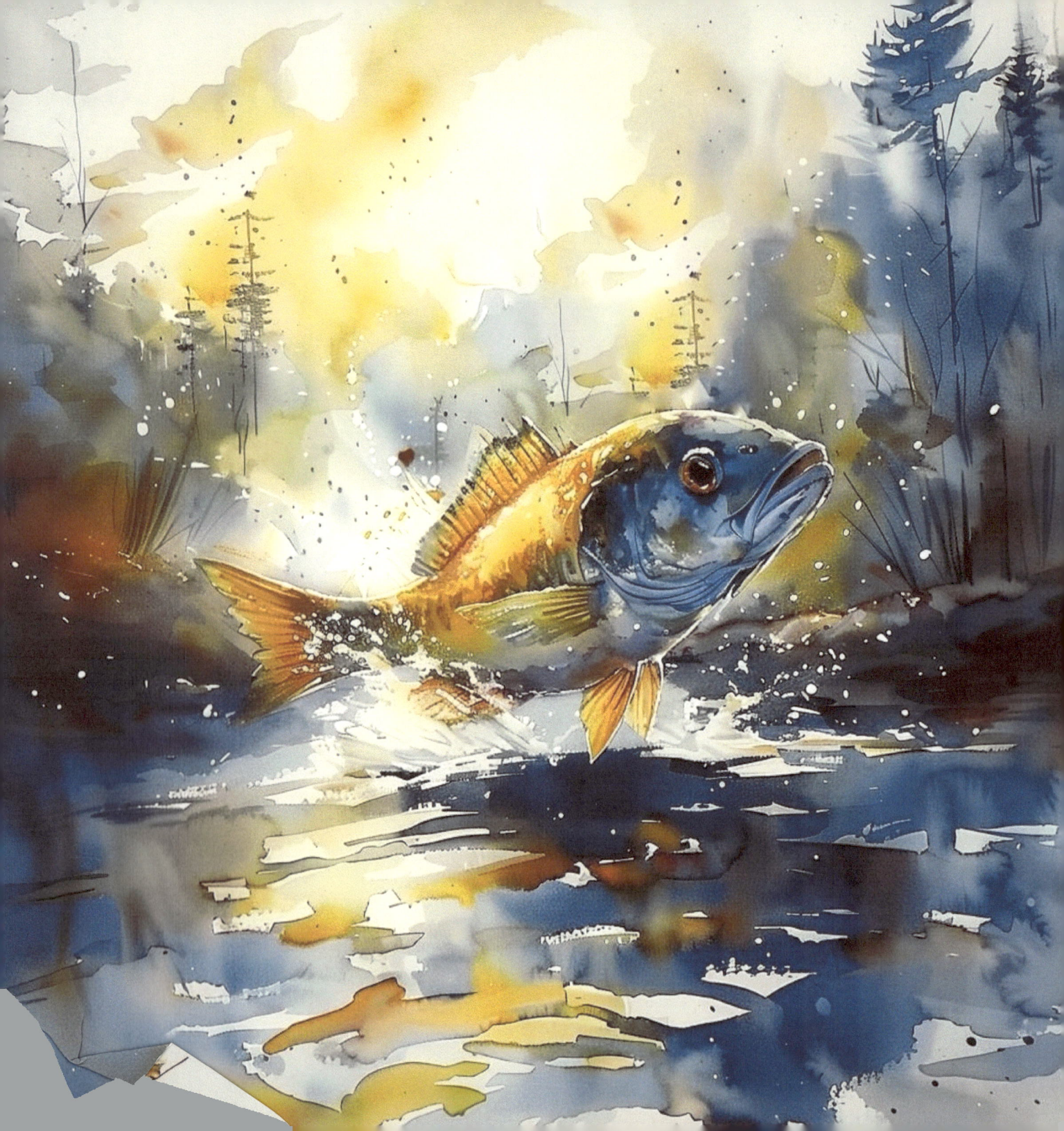

The End.

Milton Keynes UK
Ingram Content Group UK Ltd.
UKHW051356071224
451734UK00025B/119